My Favorite Ketogenic Air Freyer Recipes

Easy and Healthy Recipes to Make Unforgettable First Courses

Nolan Turner

advice. The content within this book has been derived from various sources. Please consult a licensed professional before attempting any techniques outlined in this book.

By reading this document, the reader agrees that under no circumstances is the author responsible for any losses, direct or indirect, which are incurred as a result of the use of information contained within this document, including, but not limited to, — errors, omissions, or inaccuracies.

Table of Contents

Creamy Nutmeg Cake

Prep time: 20 minutes **Cooking time:** 40 minutes
Servings: 8

Ingredients:

½ cup heavy cream

3 eggs, beaten

3 tablespoons cocoa powder

1 teaspoon vanilla extract

1 teaspoon baking powder

3 tablespoons Erythritol

1 cup almond flour

¼ teaspoon ground nutmeg

1 tablespoon avocado oil

1 teaspoon Splenda

Directions:

Mix up heavy cream and eggs in the bowl. Add cocoa powder and stir the liquid until it is smooth. After this, add vanilla extract, baking powder, Erythritol, almond flour, ground nutmeg, and avocado oil. Whisk the mixture gently and pour it in the cake mold. Then cover the cake with foil. Secure the edges of the foil. Then pierce the foil with the help of the toothpick. Preheat the air fryer to 360F. Put the cake mold in the air fryer and cook it for 40 minutes. When the cake is cooked, remove it from the air fryer and cool completely. Remove the cake from the mold and them sprinkle with Splenda.

Nutrition: calories 81, fat 6.7, fiber 1.1, carbs 3.2, protein 3.4

Parmesan Muffins

Preparation time: 5 minutes **Cooking time**: 15 minutes **Servings**: 4

Ingredients:

2 eggs, whisked Cooking spray

1 and ½ cups coconut milk 1 tablespoon baking powder

4 ounces baby spinach, chopped 2 ounces parmesan cheese, grated 3 ounces almond flour

Directions:

In a bowl, mix all the ingredients except the cooking spray and whisk really well. Grease a muffin pan that fits your air fryer with the cooking spray, divide the muffins mix, introduce the pan in the air fryer, cook at 380 degrees F for 15 minutes, divide between plates and serve.

Nutrition: calories 210, fat 12, fiber 3, carbs 5, protein 8

Cheese Eggs and Leeks

Prep time: 5 minutes **Cooking time:** 7 minutes
Servings: 2

Ingredients:

2 leeks, chopped

4 eggs, whisked

¼ cup Cheddar cheese, shredded

½ cup Mozzarella cheese, shredded

1 teaspoon avocado oil

Directions:

Preheat the air fryer to 400F. Then brush the air fryer basket with avocado oil and combine the eggs with the rest of the ingredients inside. Cook for 7 minutes and serve.

Nutrition: calories 160, fat 8.2, fiber 7.1, carbs 12.6, protein 8.6

Peppers Bowls

Preparation time: 5 minutes **Cooking time**: 20 minutes **Servings**: 4

Ingredients:

½ cup cheddar cheese, shredded 2 tablespoons chives, chopped A pinch of salt and black pepper

¼ cup coconut cream

1 cup red bell peppers, chopped Cooking spray

Directions:

In a bowl, mix all the ingredients except the cooking spray and whisk well. Pour the mix in a baking pan that fits the air fryer greased with cooking spray and place the pan in the machine. Cook at 360 degrees F for 20 minutes, divide between plates and serve for breakfast.

Nutrition: calories 220, fat 14, fiber 2, carbs 5, protein 11

Bacon Eggs

Prep time: 15 minutes **Cooking time:** 5 minutes
Servings: 2

Ingredients:

2 eggs, hard-boiled, peeled

4 bacon slices

½ teaspoon avocado oil

1 teaspoon mustard

Directions:

Preheat the air fryer to 400F. Then sprinkle the air fryer basket with avocado oil and place the bacon slices inside. Flatten them in one layer and cook for 2 minutes from each side. After this, cool the bacon to the room temperature. Wrap every egg into 2 bacon slices. Secure the eggs with toothpicks and place them in the air fryer. Cook the wrapped eggs for 1 minute at 400F.

Nutrition: calories 278, fat 20.9, fiber 0.3, carbs 1.5, protein 20

Balsamic Asparagus Salad

Preparation time: 5 minutes **Cooking time**: 10 minutes **Servings**: 4

Ingredients:

1 bunch asparagus, trimmed 1 cup baby arugula tablespoon cheddar cheese, grated 1 tablespoon balsamic vinegar

A pinch of salt and black pepper Cooking spray

Directions:

Put the asparagus in your air fryer's basket, grease with cooking spray, season with salt and pepper and cook at 360 degrees F for 10 minutes. In a bowl, mix the asparagus with the arugula and the vinegar, toss, divide between plates and serve hot with cheese sprinkled on top

Nutrition: calories 200, fat 5, fiber 1, carbs 4, protein 5

Cheddar Pancakes

Prep time: 10 minutes **Cooking time:** 7 minutes
Servings: 2

Ingredients:

2 tablespoons almond flour

¼ teaspoon baking powder

1 teaspoon Erythritol

1 teaspoon cream cheese

1 teaspoon butter, melted

2 eggs, beaten

1 bacon slice, cooked, cut into halves

1 Cheddar cheese slice

1 teaspoon sesame oil

Directions:

Make the pancake batter: in the mixing bowl mix up baking powder, almond flour, Erythritol, cream cheese, and 1 beaten egg. Preheat the air fryer to 400F. Then line the air fryer with baking paper. Pour ¼ of the pancake batter in the air fryer in the shape of pancake and cook for 1 minute. Then flip the pancake on another side and cook for 1 minute more. Repeat the same steps with the remaining pancake batter. You should get 4 pancakes. After this, brush the air fryer basket with sesame oil. Pour the remaining beaten egg in the air fryer and cook it for 3 minutes at 390F. Cut the cooked egg into 2 parts. Place the 1 half of cooked egg on the one pancake. Top it with 1 half of the bacon and second pancake.

Nutrition: calories 374, fat 31.7, fiber 3, carbs 7, protein 18.7

Green Beans Salad

Preparation time: 5 minutes : 20 minutes **Servings**: 4

Ingredients:

cups green beans, cut into medium pieces 2 cups tomatoes, cubed

Salt and black pepper to the taste 1 teaspoon hot paprika

1 tablespoons cilantro, chopped Cooking spray

Directions:

In a bowl, mix all the ingredients except the cooking spray and the cilantro and whisk them well. Grease a pan that fits the air fryer with the cooking spray, pour the green beans and tomatoes mix into the pan, sprinkle the cilantro on top, put the pan into the machine and cook at 360 degrees F for 20 minutes. Serve right away.

Nutrition: calories 222, fat 11, fiber 4, carbs 6, protein 12

Salmon and Olives

Preparation time: 5 minutes : 15 minutes **Servings**: 4

Ingredients:

1 tablespoon lemon zest, grated 1/3 cup olive oil

4 salmon fillets, boneless

1 cup green olives, pitted and sliced Juice of 2 limes

Salt and black pepper to the taste

Directions:

In a baking dish that fits your air fryer, mix all the ingredients, toss, put the pan in the fryer and cook at 370 degrees F for 15 minutes. Divide everything between plates and serve.

Nutrition: calories 204, fat 12, fiber 3, carbs 5, protein 15

Fried Crawfish

Prep time: 10 minutes **Cooking time:** 5 minutes
Servings: 4

Ingredients:

1-pound crawfish

1 tablespoon avocado oil

1 teaspoon onion powder

1 tablespoon rosemary, chopped

Directions:

Preheat the air fryer to 340F. Place the crawfish in the air fryer basket and sprinkle with avocado oil and rosemary. Add the onion powder and stir the crawfish gently. Cook the meal for 5 minutes.

Nutrition: calories 108, fat 2.1, fiber 0.5, carbs 1.2, protein 20

Lemon Shrimp and Zucchinis

Preparation time: 5 minutes   : 15 minutes

Servings: 4

Ingredients:

pound shrimp, peeled and deveined A pinch of salt and black pepper zucchinis, cut into medium cubes 1 tablespoon lemon juice

1 tablespoon olive oil

1 tablespoon garlic, minced

Directions:

In a pan that fits the air fryer, combine all the ingredients, toss, put the pan in the machine and cook at 370 degrees F for 15 minutes. Divide between plates and serve right away.

Nutrition: calories 221, fat 9, fiber 2, carbs 15, protein 11

Tuna Stuffed Avocado

Prep time: 15 minutes **Cooking time:** 12 minutes
Servings: 2

Ingredients:

1 avocado, pitted, halved

½ pound smoked tuna, boneless and shredded

1 egg, beaten

½ teaspoon salt

½ teaspoon chili powder

½ teaspoon ground nutmeg

1 teaspoon dried parsley

Cooking spray

Directions:

Scoop ½ part of the avocado meat from the avocado to get the avocado boats. Use the scooper for this step.

After this, in the mixing bowl mix up tuna and egg. Shred the mixture with the help of the fork. Add salt, chili powder, ground nutmeg, and dried parsley. Stir the tuna mixture until homogenous. Add the scooped avocado meat and mix up the mixture well. Fill the avocado boats with tuna mixture. Preheat the air fryer to 385F. Arrange the tuna boats in the air fryer basket and cook them for 12 minutes.

Nutrition: calories 400, fat 29, fiber 7.1, carbs 9.5, protein 27.4

Shrimp and Parsley Olives

Preparation time: 5 minutes **Cooking time**: 12 minutes **Servings**: 4

Ingredients:

1 pound shrimp, peeled and deveined 4 garlic clove, minced

1 cup black olives, pitted and chopped 3 tablespoons parsley

1 tablespoon olive oil

Directions:

In a pan that fits the air fryer, combine all the ingredients, toss, put the pan in the machine and cook at 380 degrees F for 12 minutes. Divide between plates and serve.

Nutrition: calories 251, fat 12, fiber 3, carbs 6, protein 15

Paprika and Cumin Shrimp

Prep time: 10 minutes **Cooking time:** 10 minutes
Servings: 4

Ingredients:

1 teaspoon chili flakes

1 teaspoon ground cumin

½ teaspoon salt

½ teaspoon dried oregano

10 oz shrimps, peeled

1 green bell pepper

2 spring onions, chopped

1 teaspoon apple cider vinegar

1 tablespoon olive oil

1 teaspoon smoked paprika

Directions:

In the mixing bowl mix up chili flakes, ground cumin, salt, dried oregano, and shrimps. Shake the mixture well. After this, preheat the air fryer to 400F. Put the spring onions in the air fryer and cook it for 3 minutes.

Meanwhile, slice the bell pepper. Add it in the air fryer and cook the vegetables for 2 minutes more. Then add shrimps and sprinkle the mixture with smoked paprika, olive oil, and apple cider vinegar. Shake it gently and cook for 5 minutes more. Transfer the cooked fajita in the serving plates.

Nutrition: calories 139, fat 5, fiber 1.3, carbs 6.6, protein 16.9

Turmeric Salmon and Cauliflower Rice

Preparation time: 5 minutes **Cooking time**: 25 minutes **Servings**: 4

Ingredients:

4 salmon fillets, boneless

Salt and black pepper to the taste 1 cup cauliflower, riced

½ cup chicken stock

1 teaspoon turmeric powder 1 tablespoon butter, melted

Directions:

In a pan that fits your air fryer, mix the cauliflower rice with the other ingredients except the salmon and toss. Arrange the salmon fillets over the cauliflower rice, put the pan in the fryer and cook at 360 degrees F for 25 minutes, flipping the fish after 15 minutes. Divide everything between plates and serve.

Nutrition: calories 241, fat 12, fiber 2, carbs 6, protein 12

Oregano Salmon

Prep time: 10 minutes **Cooking time:** 7 minutes
Servings: 2

Ingredients:

10 oz salmon fillet

1 teaspoon dried oregano

1 teaspoon sesame oil

2 oz Parmesan, grated

¼ teaspoon chili flakes

Directions:

Sprinkle the salmon fillet with dried oregano and chili flakes. Then brush it with sesame oil. Preheat the air fryer to 385F. Place the salmon in the air fryer basket and cook it for 5 minutes. Then flip the fish on another side and top with Parmesan. Cook the fish for 2 minutes more.

Nutrition: calories 301, fat 17.2, fiber 0.3, carbs 1.5, protein 36.7

Minty Trout and Pine Nuts

Preparation time: 5 minutes **Cooking time**: 16 minutes **Servings**: 4

Ingredients:

4 rainbow trout

1 cup olive oil + 3 tablespoons Juice of 1 lemon

A pinch of salt and black pepper 1 cup parsley, chopped

3 garlic cloves, minced

½ cup mint, chopped Zest of 1 lemon

1/3 pine nuts

1 avocado, peeled, pitted and roughly chopped

Directions:

Pat dry the trout, season with salt and pepper and rub with 3 tablespoons oil. Put the fish in your air fryer's basket and cook for8 minutes on each side. Divide the fish between plates and drizzle half of the lemon juice all over. In a blender, combine the rest of the oil with the remaining lemon juice, parsley, garlic, mint, lemon zest, pine nuts and the avocado and pulse well. Spread this over the trout and serve.

Nutrition: calories 240, fat 12, fiber 4, carbs 6, protein 9

Lamb and Salsa

Preparation time: 5 minutes **Cooking time**: 35 minutes **Servings**: 4

Ingredients:

1 tablespoon chipotle powder

A pinch of salt and black pepper 1 and ½ pounds lamb loin, cubed 2 tablespoons red vinegar

4 tablespoons olive oil 2 tomatoes, cubed

2 cucumbers, sliced

2 spring onions, chopped Juice of ½ lemon

¼ cup mint, chopped

Directions:

Heat up a pan that fits your air fryer with half of the oil over medium-high heat, add the lamb, stir and brown for 5 minutes. Add the chipotle powder, salt pepper and the vinegar, toss, put the pan in the air fryer and cook at 380 degrees F for 30 minutes. In a bowl, mix tomatoes with cucumbers, onions, lemon juice, mint and the rest of the oil and toss. Divide the lamb between plates, top each serving with the cucumber salsa and serve.

Nutrition: calories 284, fat 13, fiber 3, carbs 6, protein 14

Lamb Burgers

Prep time: 15 minutes **Cooking time:** 16 minutes
Servings: 2

Ingredients:

8 oz lamb, minced

½ teaspoon salt

½ teaspoon ground black pepper

½ teaspoon dried cilantro

1 tablespoon water

Cooking spray

Directions:

In the mixing bowl mix up minced lamb, salt, ground black pepper, dried cilantro, and water.

Stir the meat mixture carefully with the help of the spoon and make 2 burgers.

Preheat the air fryer to 375F.

Spray the air fryer basket with cooking spray and put the burgers inside. Cook them for 8 minutes from each side.

Nutrition: calories 219, fat 8.3, fiber 0.5, carbs 1.8, protein 32

Lime Lamb Curry

Preparation time: 5 minutes **Cooking time**: 35 minutes **Servings**: 4

Ingredients:

2 tablespoons olive oil

1   and ½ pounds lamb meat, cubed A pinch of salt and black pepper 15 ounces tomatoes, chopped Juice of 2 limes teaspoon sweet paprika 1 cup beef stock 1-inch ginger, grated 2 hot chilies, chopped red bell peppers, chopped 4 garlic cloves, minced

2   teaspoons turmeric powder 1 tablespoon green curry paste

Directions:

Heat up a pan that fits your air fryer with the oil over medium heat, add the meat and brown for 5 minutes. Add the rest of the ingredients, toss, put the pan in the fryer and cook at 380 degrees F for 30 minutes. Divide everything into bowls and serve.

Nutrition: calories 284, fat 12, fiber 3, carbs 5, protein 16

Lamb Sausages

Prep time: 25 minutes **Cooking time:** 10 minutes
Servings: 4

Ingredients:

4 sausage links

12 oz ground lamb

1 teaspoon minced garlic

½ teaspoon onion powder

1 teaspoon dried parsley

½ teaspoon salt

1 teaspoon ghee

½ teaspoon ground ginger

1 tablespoon sesame oil

Directions:

In the mixing bowl mix up ground lamb, minced garlic, onion powder, dried parsley, salt, and ground ginger.

Then fill the sausage links with the ground lamb mixture. Secure the ends of the sausages. Brush the air fryer basket with sesame oil from inside and put the sausages. Then sprinkle the sausages with ghee. Cook the lamb sausages for 10 minutes at 400F. Flip them on another side after 5 minutes of cooking.

Nutrition: calories 201, fat 10.7, fiber 0.1, carbs 0.7, protein 24

Lamb and Vinaigrette

Preparation time: 10 minutes **Cooking time:** 30 minutes **Servings**: 4

Ingredients:

4 lamb loin slices

A pinch of salt and black pepper 3 garlic cloves, minced

2 teaspoons thyme, chopped 2 tablespoons olive oil

1/3 cup parsley, chopped

1/3 cup sun-dried tomatoes, chopped 2 tablespoons balsamic vinegar

2 tablespoons water

Directions:

In a blender, combine all the ingredients except the lamb slices and pulse well. In a bowl, mix the lamb with the tomato vinaigrette and toss well.

Put the lamb in your air fryer's basket and cook at 380 degrees F for 15 minutes on each side. Divide everything between plates and serve.

Nutrition: calories 273, fat 13, fiber 4, carbs 6, protein 17

Ginger and Turmeric Lamb

Prep time: 15 minutes **Cooking time:** 25 minutes
Servings: 4

Ingredients:

16 oz rack of lamb

1 teaspoon ginger paste

½ teaspoon ground ginger

½ teaspoon salt

½ teaspoon ground paprika

¼ teaspoon ground turmeric

1 tablespoon butter, melted

1 teaspoon olive oil

Directions:

In the mixing bowl mix up ground ginger, ginger paste, salt, ground paprika, turmeric, butter, and olive oil. Then brush the rack of lamb with the butter mixture and put it in the air fryer. Cook the rack of lamb for 25 minutes at 380F.

Nutrition: calories 229, fat 14.2, fiber 0.2, carbs 0.6, protein 23.2

Parmesan Lamb Cutlets

Preparation time: 5 minutes **Cooking time**: 30 minutes **Servings**: 4

Ingredients:

8 lamb cutlets

A pinch of salt and black pepper 3 tablespoons mustard

3 tablespoons olive oil

½ cup coconut flakes

¼ cup parmesan, grated

2 tablespoons parsley, chopped 2 tablespoons chives, chopped

1 tablespoon rosemary, chopped

Directions:

In a bowl, mix the lamb cutlets with all the ingredients except the parmesan and the coconut flakes and toss well. Dredge the cutlets in parmesan and coconut flakes, put them in your air fryer's basket and cook at 390 degrees F for 15 minutes on each side. Divide between plates and serve.

Nutrition: calories 284, fat 13, fiber 3, carbs 6, protein 17

Mint and Rosemary Lamb

Prep time: 2 hours **Cooking time:** 35 minutes

Servings: 2

Ingredients:

12 oz leg of lamb, boneless

1 teaspoon dried rosemary

½ teaspoon dried mint

1 garlic clove, diced

½ teaspoon salt

¼ teaspoon ground black pepper

1 teaspoon apple cider vinegar

1 tablespoon olive oil

Directions:

In the mixing bowl mix up dried rosemary, mint, diced garlic, salt, ground black pepper, apple cider vinegar, and olive oil. Then rub the leg of lamb with the spice mixture and leave for 2 hours to marinate. After this, preheat the air fryer to 400F. Put the leg of lamb in the air fryer and sprinkle with all remaining spice mixture. Cook the meal for 25 minutes. Then flip the meat on another side and cook it for 10 minutes more.

Nutrition: calories 382, fat 19.6, fiber 0.4, carbs 1.1, protein 47.9

Lamb and Scallion Balls

Preparation time: 5 minutes **Cooking time:** 30 minutes **Servings**: 4

Ingredients: and ½ pounds lamb, ground 1 scallion, chopped

A pinch of salt and black pepper

½ cup pine nuts, toasted and chopped 1 tablespoon thyme, chopped garlic cloves, minced 1 tablespoon olive oil 1 egg, whisked

Directions:

In a bowl, mix the lamb with the rest of the ingredients except the oil, stir well and shape medium meatballs out of this mix. Grease the meatballs with the oil, put them in your air fryer's basket and cook at 380 degrees F for 15 minutes on each side. Divide between plates and serve with a side salad.

Nutrition: calories 287, fat 12, fiber 3, carbs 6, protein 17

Spicy Buttered Steaks

Prep time: 15 minutes **Cooking time:** 17 minutes
Servings: 4

Ingredients:

1-pound beef rib eye steak, bone-in (4 steaks)

1 tablespoon butter

1 teaspoon garlic, diced

½ teaspoon lime zest, grated

½ teaspoon ground paprika

½ teaspoon ground ginger

½ teaspoon chipotle powder

1 teaspoon salt

½ teaspoon chili flakes

Directions:

Rub the meat steaks with garlic, lime zest, ground paprika, ground ginger, chipotle powder, salt, and chili flakes, then melt the butter and brush the meat with it. Put the steaks in the air fryer and cook them for 17 minutes at 400F. Flip the meat on another side after 10 minutes of cooking.

Nutrition: calories 287, fat 22.9, fiber 1.1, carbs 3, protein 15.7

Moroccan Lamb and Garlic

Preparation time: 5 minutes **Cooking time**: 30 minutes **Servings**: 4

Ingredients:

8 lamb cutlets

A pinch of salt and black pepper 4 tablespoons olive oil

½ cup mint leaves 6 garlic cloves

1 tablespoon cumin, ground 1 tablespoon coriander seeds Zest of 2 lemons, grated

3 tablespoons lemon juice

Directions:

In a blender, combine all the ingredients except the lamb and pulse well. Rub the lamb cutlets with this mix, place them in your air fryer's basket and cook at 380 degrees F for 15 minutes on each side. Serve with a side salad.

Nutrition: calories 284, fat 13, fiber 3, carbs 5, protein 15

Ribs and Chimichuri Mix

Prep time: 10 minutes **Cooking time:** 35 minutes
Servings: 4

Ingredients:

1-pound pork baby back ribs, boneless

2 tablespoons chimichuri sauce

½ teaspoon salt

Directions:

Sprinkle the ribs with salt and brush with chimichuri sauce. Then preheat the air fryer to 365F. Put the pork ribs in the air fryer and cook for 35 minutes.

Nutrition: calories 504, fat 43.3, fiber 1, carbs 1, protein 25.9

Roasted Lamb

Preparation time: 5 minutes **Cooking time**: 30 minutes **Servings**: 4

Ingredients:

8 lamb cutlets

2 tablespoons olive oil

A pinch of salt and black pepper 2 tablespoons rosemary, chopped 2 garlic cloves, minced

A pinch of cayenne pepper

Directions:

In a bowl, mix the lamb with the rest of the ingredients and rub well. Put the lamb in the fryer's basket and cook at 380 degrees F for 30 minutes, flipping them halfway. Divide the cutlets between plates and serve.

Nutrition: calories 274, fat 12, fiber 3, carbs 5, protein 15

Peppermint Lamb

Prep time: 15 minutes **Cooking time:** 12 minutes
Servings: 4

Ingredients:

1-pound lamb chops

2 oz celery ribs, chopped

½ teaspoon lemon zest, grated

½ teaspoon garlic, minced

½ teaspoon peppermint

1 tablespoon ghee

½ teaspoon ground black pepper

1 teaspoon olive oil

Directions:

Put the celery ribs in the blender. Add lemon zest, garlic, peppermint, ghee, ground black pepper, and olive oil.

Pulse the mixture for 1-2 minutes. Then carefully rub the lamb chops with blended mixture and put the meat in the air fryer. Cook the lamb chops for 6 minutes from each side at 400F.

Nutrition: calories 314, fat 17.5, fiber 0.9, carbs 3.4, protein 34.7

Mustard Chives and Basil Lamb

Preparation time: 10 minutes **Cooking time**: 30 minutes **Servings**: 4

Ingredients:

8 lamb cutlets

A pinch of salt and black pepper A drizzle of olive oil

2 garlic cloves, minced

¼ cup mustard

1 tablespoon chives, chopped 1 tablespoon basil, chopped

1 tablespoon oregano, chopped 1 tablespoon mint chopped

Directions:

In a bowl, mix the lamb with the rest of the ingredients and rub well. Put the cutlets in your air fryer's basket and cook at 380 degrees F for 15 minutes on each side. Divide between plates and serve with a side salad.

Nutrition: calories 284, fat 13, fiber 3, carbs 6, protein 14

Lamb with Paprika Cilantro Sauce

Preparation time: 5 minutes **Cooking time**: 30 minutes **Servings**: 4

Ingredients:

1 pound lamb, cubed 1 cup coconut cream

3 tablespoons sweet paprika 2 tablespoons olive oil

2 tablespoons cilantro, chopped Salt and black pepper to the taste

Directions:

Heat up a pan that fits your air fryer with the oil over medium-high heat, add the meat and brown for 5 minutes. Add the rest of the ingredients, toss, put the pan in the air fryer and cook at 380 degrees F for 25 minutes. Divide everything into bowls and serve.

Nutrition: calories 287, fat 13, fiber 2, carbs 6, protein 12

Tomatoes Frittata

Preparation time: 5 minutes **Cooking time**: 20 minutes **Servings**: 4

Ingredients:

4 eggs, whisked

1 pound cherry tomatoes, halved 1 tablespoon parsley, chopped Cooking spray

1 tablespoon cheddar, grated Salt and black pepper to the taste

Directions:

Put the tomatoes in the air fryer's basket, cook at 360 degrees F for 5 minutes and transfer them to the baking pan that fits the machine greased with cooking spray. In a bowl, mix the eggs with the remaining ingredients, whisk, pour over the tomatoes an cook at 360 degrees F for 15 minutes. Serve right away for breakfast.

Nutrition: calories 230, fat 14, fiber 3, carbs 5, protein 11

French Frittata

Prep time: 10 minutes **Cooking time:** 18 minutes
Servings: 3

Ingredients:

3 eggs

1 tablespoon heavy cream

1 teaspoon Herbs de Provence

1 teaspoon almond butter, softened

2 oz Provolone cheese, grated

Directions:

Crack the eggs in the bowl and add heavy cream. Whisk the liquid with the help of the hand whisker. Then add herbs de Provence and grated cheese. Stir the egg liquid gently. Preheat the air fryer to 365F. Then grease the air fryer basket with almond butter. Pour the egg liquid in the air fryer basket and cook it for 18 minutes. When the frittata is cooked, cool it to the room temperature and then cut into servings.

Nutrition: calories 179, fat 14.3, fiber 0.5, carbs 1.9, protein 11.6

Paprika Zucchini Spread

Preparation time: 5 minutes **Cooking time**: 15 minutes **Servings**: 4

Ingredients:

4 zucchinis, roughly chopped 1 tablespoon sweet paprika

Salt and black pepper to the taste 1 tablespoon butter, melted

Directions:

Grease a baking pan that fits the Air Fryer with the butter, add all the ingredients, toss, and cook at 360 degrees F for 15 minutes. Transfer to a blender, pulse well, divide into bowls and serve for breakfast.

Nutrition: calories 240, fat 14, fiber 2, carbs 5, protein 11

Dill Egg Rolls

Prep time: 10 minutes **Cooking time:** 4 minutes
Servings: 4

Ingredients:

2 eggs, hard-boiled, peeled

1 tablespoon cream cheese

1 tablespoon fresh dill, chopped

1 teaspoon ground black pepper

4 wontons wrap

1 egg white, whisked

1 teaspoon sesame oil

Directions:

Chop the eggs and mix them up with cream cheese, dill, and ground black pepper. Then place the egg mixture on the wonton wraps and roll them into the rolls. Brush every roll with whisked egg white. After this, preheat the air fryer to 395F and brush the air fryer basket with sesame oil.

Arrange the egg rolls in the hot air fryer and cook them for 2 minutes from each side or until the rolls are golden brown.

Nutrition: calories 81 fat 4.4, fiber 0.4, carbs 5.7, protein 4.9

Parsley Omelet

Preparation time: 5 minutes **Cooking time**: 15 minutes **Servings**: 4

Ingredients: 4 eggs,

whisked tablespoon parsley,

chopped

½ teaspoons cheddar cheese, shredded 1 avocado, peeled, pitted and cubed Cooking spray

Directions:

In a bowl, mix all the ingredients except the cooking spray and whisk well. Grease a baking pan that fits the Air Fryer with the cooking spray, pour the omelet mix, spread, introduce the pan in the machine and cook at 370 degrees F for 15 minutes. Serve for breakfast.

Nutrition: calories 240, fat 13, fiber 4, carbs 6, protein 9

Hard-Boiled Eggs

Prep time: 8 minutes **Cooking time:** 16 minutes

Servings: 2

Ingredients:

4 eggs

¼ teaspoon salt

Directions:

Place the eggs in the air fryer and cook them for 16 minutes at 250F. When the eggs are cooked, cool them in the ice water. After this, peel the eggs and cut into halves. Sprinkle the eggs with salt.

Nutrition: calories 126, fat 8.8, fiber 0, carbs 0.7, protein 11.1

Spinach Spread

Preparation time: 5 minutes **Cooking time**: 10 minutes **Servings**: 4

Ingredients: tablespoons coconut cream 3 cups spinach leaves

2 tablespoons cilantro

2 tablespoons bacon, cooked and crumbled Salt and black pepper to the taste

Directions:

In a pan that fits the air fryer, combine all the ingredients except the bacon, put the pan in the machine and cook at 360 degrees F for 10 minutes. Transfer to a blender, pulse well, divide into bowls and serve with bacon sprinkled on top.

Nutrition: calories 200, fat 4, fiber 2, carbs 4, protein 4

Peppers Cups

Prep time: 10 minutes **Cooking time:** 12 minutes
Servings: 12

Ingredients:

6 green bell peppers

12 egg

½ teaspoon ground black pepper

½ teaspoon chili flakes

Directions:

Cut the green bell peppers into halves and remove the seeds. Then crack the eggs in every bell pepper half and sprinkle with ground black pepper and chili flakes. After this, preheat the air fryer to 395F. Put the green bell pepper halves in the air fryer (cook for 2-3 halves per one time of cooking). Cook the egg peppers for 4 minutes. Repeat the same steps with remaining egg peppers.

Nutrition: calories 82, fat 4.5, fiber 0.8, carbs 4.9, protein 6.2

Chives Spinach Frittata

Preparation time: 5 minutes **Cooking time**: 20 minutes **Servings:** 4

Ingredients:

1 tablespoon chives, chopped 1 eggplant, cubed

8 ounces spinach, torn Cooking spray

6 eggs, whisked

Salt and black pepper to the taste

Directions:

In a bowl, mix the eggs with the rest of the ingredients except the cooking spray and whisk well. Grease a pan that fits your air fryer with the cooking spray, pour the frittata mix, spread and put the pan in the machine. Cook at 380 degrees F for 20 minutes, divide between plates and serve for breakfast.

Nutrition: calories 240, fat 8, fiber 3, carbs 6, protein 12

Mozzarella Rolls

Prep time: 15 minutes **Cooking time:** 6 minutes
Servings: 6

Ingredients:

6 wonton wrappers

1 tablespoon keto tomato sauce

½ cup Mozzarella, shredded

1 oz pepperoni, chopped

1 egg, beaten

Cooking spray

Directions:

In the big bowl mix up together shredded Mozzarella, pepperoni, and tomato sauce. When the mixture is homogenous transfer it on the wonton wraps. Wrap the wonton wraps in the shape of sticks. Then brush them with beaten eggs. Preheat the air fryer to 400F. Spray the air fryer basket with cooking spray. Put the pizza sticks in the air fryer and cook them for 3 minutes from each side.

Nutrition: calories 65, fat 3.5, fiber 0.2, carbs 4.9, protein 3.5

Chili Tomato Pork

Prep time: 15 minutes **Cooking time:** 15 minutes **Servings:** 3

Ingredients:

12 oz pork tenderloin

1 tablespoon grain mustard

1 tablespoon swerve

1 tablespoon keto tomato sauce

1 teaspoon chili pepper, grinded

¼ teaspoon garlic powder

1 tablespoon olive oil

Directions:

In the mixing bowl mix up grain mustard, swerve, tomato sauce, chili pepper, garlic powder, and olive oil. Rub the pork tenderloin with mustard mixture generously and leave for 5-10 minutes to marinate. Meanwhile, preheat the air fryer to 370F. Put the marinated pork tenderloin in the air fryer baking pan. Then insert the baking pan in the preheated air fryer and cook the meat for 15 minutes. Cool the cooked meat to the room temperature and slice it into the servings.

Nutrition: calories 212, fat 9, fiber 0.2, carbs 6.4, protein 29.8

Chili Pork

Preparation time: 5 minutes **Cooking time**: 25 minutes **Servings:** 4

Ingredients:

2 teaspoons chili paste 2 garlic cloves, minced 4 pork chops

1 shallot, chopped

1 and ½ cups coconut milk 2 tablespoons olive oil tablespoons coconut aminos Salt and black pepper to the taste

Directions:

In a pan that fits your air fryer, mix the pork the rest of the ingredients, toss, introduce the pan in the fryer and cook at 400 degrees F for 25 minutes, shaking the fryer halfway. Divide everything into bowls and serve.

Nutrition: calories 267, fat 12, fiber 4, carbs 6, protein 18

Cilantro Beef Meatballs

Prep time: 20 minutes **Cooking time:** 7 minutes
Servings: 4

Ingredients:

1 cup ground beef

3 oz Cheddar cheese, shredded

1 tablespoons flax meal

1 teaspoon fresh cilantro, chopped

1 garlic clove, diced

1 chili pepper, chopped

1 egg, beaten

1 teaspoon ground coriander

¼ cup scallions, diced

½ teaspoon ground black pepper

1 teaspoon avocado oil

Directions:

Put the ground beef in the bowl and mix it up with flax meal, cilantro, garlic clove, chili pepper, egg, ground coriander, diced onion, and ground black pepper. When the mixture is homogenous, add shredded Cheddar cheese and stir the mixture with the help of the spoon. Make the small meatballs from the ground beef mixture. Then preheat the air fryer to 380F. Brush the air fryer basket with avocado oil from inside and arrange the prepared meatballs in one layer. Cook them for 7 minutes or until the meatballs are light brown.

Nutrition: calories 180, fat 13, fiber 0.8, carbs 2.1, protein 13.8

Basil Pork

Preparation time: 5 minutes **Cooking time**: 25 minutes **Servings**: 4

Ingredients: pork

chops

A pinch of salt and black pepper 2 teaspoons basil, dried

2 tablespoons olive oil

½ teaspoon chili powder

Directions:

In a pan that fits your air fryer, mix all the ingredients, toss, introduce in the fryer and cook at 400 degrees F for 25 minutes. Divide everything between plates and serve.

Nutrition: calories 274, fat 13, fiber 4, carbs 6, protein 18

Pork and Asparagus

Preparation time: 5 minutes **Cooking time**: 35 minutes **Servings:** 4

Ingredients: pounds pork loin, boneless and cubed

¾ cup beef stock tablespoons

olive oil tablespoons keto

tomato sauce

1 pound asparagus, trimmed and halved

½ tablespoon oregano, chopped Salt and black pepper to the taste

Directions:

Heat up a pan that fits your air fryer with the oil over medium heat, add the pork, toss and brown for 5 minutes. Add the rest of the ingredients, toss a bit, put the pan in the fryer and cook at 380 degrees F for 30 minutes. Divide everything between plates and serve.

Nutrition: calories 287, fat 13, fiber 4, carbs 6, protein 18

Wrapped Pork

Prep time: 20 minutes **Cooking time:** 16 minutes
Servings: 2

Ingredients:

8 oz pork tenderloin

4 bacon slices

½ teaspoon salt

1 teaspoon olive oil

½ teaspoon chili powder

Directions:

Sprinkle the pork tenderloin with salt and chili powder. Then wrap it in the bacon slices and sprinkle with olive oil. Secure the bacon with toothpicks if needed. After this, preheat the air fryer to 375F. Put the wrapped pork tenderloin in the air fryer and cook it for 7 minutes. After this, carefully flip the meat on another side and cook it for 9 minutes more. When the meat is cooked, remove the toothpicks from it (if the toothpicks were used) and slice the meat.

Nutrition: calories 390, fat 22.3, fiber 0.2, carbs 0.9, protein 43.8

Cinnamon Ghee Pork Chops

Preparation time: 5 minutes **Cooking time**: 35 minutes **Servings**: 4

Ingredients:

4 pork chops, bone-in

A pinch of salt and black pepper 2 and ½ tablespoons ghee, melted

½ teaspoon chipotle chili powder

½ teaspoon cinnamon powder

½ teaspoon garlic powder

½ teaspoon allspice

1 teaspoon coconut sugar

Directions:

Rub the pork chops with all the other ingredients, put them in your air fryer's basket and cook at 380 degrees

F for 35 minutes. Divide the chops between plates and serve with a side salad.

Nutrition: calories 287, fat 14, fiber 4, carbs 7, protein 18

Creamy Pork Chops

Prep time: 15 minutes **Cooking time:** 10 minutes
Servings: 4

Ingredients:

2 pork chops

¼ cup coconut flakes

3 tablespoons almond flour

½ teaspoon salt

½ teaspoon dried parsley

1 egg, beaten

1 tablespoon heavy cream

1 teaspoon butter, melted

Directions:

Cut every pork chops into 2 chops. Then sprinkle them
with salt and dried parsley. After this, in the mixing bowl

mix up coconut flakes and almond flour. In the separated bowl mix up egg, heavy cream, and melted butter. Coat the pork chops in the almond flour mixture and them dip in the egg mixture. Repeat the same steps one more time. Then coat the pork chops in the remaining almond flour mixture. Place the meat in the air fryer basket. Cook the pork chops for 10 minutes at 400F. Flip them on another side after 5 minutes of cooking.

Nutrition: calories 303, fat 25.6, fiber 2.7, carbs 5.5, protein 15.1

Shoulder

Prep time: 20 minutes **Cooking time:** 20 minutes
Servings: 4

Ingredients:

1-pound pork shoulder, boneless

3 spring onions, chopped

1 teaspoon dried dill

1 teaspoon keto tomato sauce

1 tablespoon water

1 teaspoon salt

2 tablespoons sesame oil

1 teaspoon ground black pepper

½ teaspoon garlic powder

Directions:

In the shallow bowl mix up salt, ground black pepper, and garlic powder. Then add dried dill. Sprinkle the pork shoulder with a spice mixture from each side. Then in the separated bowl, mix up tomato sauce, water, and sesame oil. Brush the meat with the tomato mixture. Then place it on the foil. Add spring onions. Wrap the pork shoulder. Preheat the air fryer to 395F. Put the wrapped pork shoulder in the air fryer basket and cook it for 20 minutes. Let the cooked meat rest for 5-10 minutes and then discard the foil.

Nutrition: calories 401, fat 31.1, fiber 0.5, carbs 2.3, protein 26.8

Coconut Walnuts

Preparation time: 5 minutes **Cooking time**: 40 minutes **Servings**: 12

Ingredients:

1 and ¼ cups almond flour 1 cup swerve

1 cup butter, melted

½ cup coconut cream

1 and ½ cups coconut, flaked 1 egg yolk

¾ cup walnuts, chopped

½ teaspoon vanilla extract

Directions:

In a bowl, mix the flour with half of the swerve and half of the butter, stir well and press this on the bottom of a baking pan that fits the air fryer.

Introduce this in the air fryer and cook at 350 degrees F for 15 minutes. Meanwhile, heat up a pan with the rest of the butter over medium heat, add the remaining swerve and the rest of the ingredients, whisk, cook for 12 minutes, take off the heat and cool down. Spread this well over the crust, put the pan in the air fryer again and cook at 350 degrees F for 25 minutes. Cool down, cut into bars and serve.

Nutrition: calories 182, fat 12, fiber 2, carbs 4, protein 4

Buttery Muffins

Prep time: 15 minutes **Cooking time:** 10 minutes
Servings: 2

Ingredients:

1 teaspoon of cocoa powder

2 tablespoons coconut flour

2 teaspoons swerve

½ teaspoon vanilla extract

2 teaspoons almond butter, melted

¼ teaspoon baking powder

1 teaspoon apple cider vinegar

¼ teaspoon ground cinnamon

Directions:

In the mixing bowl mix up cocoa powder, coconut flour, swerve, vanilla extract, almond butter, baking powder, and apple cider vinegar. Then add ground cinnamon and stir the mixture with the help of the spoon until it is smooth. Pour the brownie mixture in the muffin molds and leave for 10 minutes to rest. Meanwhile, preheat the air fryer to 365F. Put the muffins in the air fryer basket and cook them for 10 minutes. Then remove the cooked brownie muffins from the air fryer and cool them completely.

Nutrition: calories 145, fat 10.4, fiber 5, carbs 10.7, protein 5.1

Lemon Butter Bars

Preparation time: 10 minutes **Cooking time**: 35 minutes **Servings**: 8

Ingredients:

½ cup butter, melted 1 cup erythritol and

¾ cups almond flour 3 eggs, whisked

Zest of 1 lemon, grated Juice of 3 lemons

Directions:

In a bowl, mix 1 cup flour with half of the erythritol and the butter, stir well and press into a baking dish that fits the air fryer lined with parchment paper. Put the dish in your air fryer and cook at 350 degrees F for 10 minutes. Meanwhile, in a bowl, mix the rest of the flour with the remaining erythritol and the other ingredients and whisk well. Spread this over the crust, put the dish in the air fryer once more and cook at 350 degrees F for 25 minutes. Cool down, cut into bars and serve.

Nutrition: calories 210, fat 12, fiber 1, carbs 4, protein 8

Nut Bars

Prep time: 15 minutes **Cooking time:** 30 minutes
Servings: 10

Ingredients:

½ cup coconut oil, softened

1 teaspoon baking powder

1 teaspoon lemon juice

1 cup almond flour

½ cup coconut flour

3 tablespoons Erythritol

1 teaspoon vanilla extract

2 eggs, beaten

2 oz hazelnuts, chopped

1 oz macadamia nuts, chopped

Cooking spray **Directions:**

In the mixing bowl mix up coconut oil and baking powder. Add lemon juice, almond flour, coconut flour, Erythritol, vanilla extract, and eggs. Stir the mixture until it is smooth or use the immersion blender for this step. Then add hazelnuts and macadamia nuts. Stir the mixture until homogenous. After this, preheat the air fryer to 325F. Line the air fryer basket with baking paper. Then pour the nut mixture in the air fryer basket and flatten it well with the help of the spatula. Cook the mixture for 30 minutes. Then cool the mixture well and cut it into the serving bars.

Nutrition: calories 208, fat 19.8, fiber 3.5, carbs 9.5, protein 4

www.ingramcontent.com/pod-product-compliance
Lightning Source LLC
Chambersburg PA
CBHW050759030426
42336CB00012B/1869